# 17 Day Diet For Beginners:

## Lose Weight, Lose Body Fat, Get Flat Belly and Slim Body in a Healthy Way Fast

By

Brittany Samons

# Table of Contents

17 Day Diet For Beginners: Lose Weight, Lose Body Fat, Get Flat Belly and Slim Body in a Healthy Way Fast

By Brittany Samons

First Published, 2015

Printed in the United States of America

# Introduction

Being overweight is getting very common nowadays. The number of obese people is increasing quickly, many nutritionist and dieticians blame fast food for it as people eat more from fast food restaurants. Obesity itself is the major cause for many diseases such as heart problems, blood pressure issues, cholesterol problems etc. The choice is with the people whether they want to live a healthy life or just go along the way they are living. People who want to change their eating habits can still do it. All they need is the will power and a good diet plan.

17 day diet plan was developed to help overweight people to lose their weight. The main goal of this diet plan is not only to help obese people to start losing the weight, but also to remove the health problems that are usually associated with the big weight.

There is a lot of misconception and lack of knowledge among the people regarding the dieting. This is the reason that they start crash dieting in the initial stage of dieting which is very bad for the help. They think it would help to reduce the weight soon but the reality is quite contrary. It effects health very badly and many people start having problems such as fatigue, dizziness, weakness etc. This book will help such beginners as it will tell what they should do and how to diet to get the most effective results.

# Chapter 1. Cycle of 17 Day Diet Plan

This diet plan helps to reduce the weight and shed the extra pounds you have gained. This kind of plan is divided into the seventeen day cycles so that the follower does not get bored and keeps on following it as it does result in positive results. After the passage of seventeen days you will enter a new cycle. It has four cycles in total which are explained below.

The first cycle is the acceleration, in this the focus is on to improve the digestion and reduce sugar level from blood so that more fat can be burned. This is cycle you are supposed to eat low processed food, more lean protein, less fat, more vegetables, low carb and less starchy vegetables along with low fat protein. This stage is to start the program and set the goals to burn the fats and not letting extra fats to be stored in the body. This has to be followed for seventeen days, then you move to the second cycle.

Second cycle is based on the activation of the metabolism rather resetting it in a pace that will help in reducing the weight, in which the consumption of calories is adjusted which leads to the burning of the fats more. Starch can be added in this stage so one switches between cycle one and two. It also lasts for seventeen days in total.

The third cycle is about achieving. This cycle helps to you start developing the eating habits which are good for your health and it also leads you towards your future goal. Some new foods are introduced in this stage and intake of proteins in reduced. The time period of this cycle is also seventeen days.

Last cycle is about arriving; this one has claimed that one remains at their goal weight. It is more about maintaining what you have achieved and not letting your body to gain more again. In this stage you are allowed to eat the food you desire on the weekend and eat the healthy diet during the weekdays. The healthy diet is the same that is in the cycle one, two and three.

When you reach the fourth cycle in which you have achieved the goal then you should acknowledge you accomplishment. This does not mean that you have to leave what you started. So, after this stage you are advised to jump back to the first stages to keep the cycle going. The efforts are required to maintain the developed schedule. This cycle should be followed to remain healthy and fit. This overall diet plan is very flexible and it can be sustained overtime. It is not restricted to some special group of people or places. The reason that it should be followed is that it recommends the healthy diet with carbohydrates, healthy fats and it is against the processed food and fried food. All the stages in the cycle should be followed properly to get the desired results.

**The Exercise**

One thing which is very important in this diet plan is the exercise. If you want to reduce weight and remain healthy then you will need to be little more active and exercise. For the ones who had just begun this cycle are required to do 17 minute exercise daily. Exercise does not mean you have to do something tough. It can be as simple as a seventeen minute walk or light exercise which can be learned from the videos or from available DVD. However, the plan has to change as you progress into different stages of the 17 day diet plan. In the first two cycles the requirement remains at 17 minute exercise. It changes when you enter third cycle in which you are required to do 40-60 minute aerobic exercise. In the fourth stage you should keep on exercising during the week days in the same routine but on the weekends try to extend the time till an hour.

# Chapter 3. The Principles of The Diet

It is true that everyone has a different functioning body and things which suit one person may not bring wonderful results for another but there are some principles in the diet plan which are universal. It is also confirmed by many nutritionists who have varying experience. Many people who has just start their diet may not know about them. It is very important for them to know about it because it will lead to a healthy body which they would love. These principles would help to create a healthy diet plan and they would be able to follow it.

Following are among the most important principles:

**Having a Balanced Diet**

It is the law of nature to use everything in right quantity as excessive use of anything will lead to negative results. Unbalanced diet leads the people to eat one type of food more and other food rich of nutrients which is essential for the body less so their bodies lack the right amount of important nutrients. One thinks that he/she will lose weight but unbalanced diet can lead to weight gain rather than the loss. Before creating the plan keeps it in mind to include various kind of food especially vegetables to consume each kind of nutrients like proteins, vitamins, fiber etc. This will ensure the proper functioning of the body and it will remain healthy.

**The Timing of the Nutrients**

It is very important to eat the right thing at the right time to get best results in dieting. To optimize the body composition it is essential when we eat along with what we eat. Generally, people tend to skip the breakfast which is not a wise thing to do because it leads to more weight gain. Breakfast is very important for the body as it is the initial fuel needed for kick start our body in the morning. As the day passes, less should be eaten and dinner should be light as compared to the other meals. During the day one can eat smaller meals throughout the day with proper gap. A study has shown that people eat three times a day and the meals consumed in them are very large. So, eating at proper time matters most.

**Monitor Yourself**

When you plan to diet then keep in mind that you have to keep in track how many times you eat in a day and how much food is consumed during the meals. There should be check and balance. If you will pay proper attention to what you are eating then you can reduce the calorie intake as you would know which kind of food has most or least calorie. Studies have shown that such people tend to lose more because they know what they are eating and how much calories they are consuming in a day. They are conscious about their diets which help to reduce the weight. After a specific time period, say a couple of weeks after you started dieting, do weigh yourself because it would motivate you when you will see the positive result with your own eyes.

**Restrict Selective Food**

The kind of foods that are forbidden to eat in a diet plan vary from one plan to another. Some of them are high in proteins and forbids food that have fats or the ones high in carbohydrates would discourage the use of proteins in large amount. So it depends on what kind of plan you are following. It is essential to avoid some types of food to make the diet plan work such as food with high rate of fats should not be consumed because they tend to increase the weight. Avoid any kind of food that increases the weight such as the sweets, processed foods and animal food. One thing should be kept in mind that do not take the restrictions to the extreme because sometimes it can lead to malnutrition so you can have a cheat day now and then when you can eat whatever you want to satisfy your cravings.

**Consume Low Calorie**

There is concept of calorie density which you should be aware of. It means the calorie a food contains in one unit of its volume. When consuming meals, be aware of foods with high calorie density as they have high number of calories in them and a very small intake of such foods leads to large intake of calorie without your knowledge. The foods which have lots of water and fiber in it tend to have the least or close to none calorie density so looks out and consumes such food more. To reduce weight eats the food with less calorie density.

## Be Consistent

Humans are impatient by nature. They want results immediately and it is very hard for them to stick to one thing for a long time. When you think of dieting or start a diet plan, then are patient and consistent. You can only see the positive result if you will follow the plan strictly for a long period of time. Keep the consistent plan throughout the year to reduce weight.

## Remain Motivated

People always wonder how others reduce weight easily while they have to struggle. The reason is that they remain motivated that they can do it; they do not give up easily or quickly. This is what helps them to follow the plan because they know the results would be very satisfying. Do not blame your genes for it, everyone can do it, all you need is a little speck of motivation to keep you going. Do not expect wonders to happen overnight, let the magic of dieting work its way through with some time.

## Benefits of Following The Basic Principles

All the principles explained above have many benefits that will help you through the seventeen day diet plan which can be extended if you feel you are seeing positive result in your body. Basically these principles tell the main points on which one should ponder before trying out the diet because they are the reason which lead to the healthy life. They are interlinked with each other and one cannot be achieved by ignoring some of them and adopting others.

These lead to the healthy living and weight loss.

You get to know what kind of food is good for you and what ones should be consumed less. It would increase your knowledge because it is very important to know what you are putting inside your body. A healthy living will lead to a successful life because you would be able to achieve what you want without serious health issues that restrict you to certain activities while forbidding others. A person consuming the balanced diet would know when to eat and how much to eat, what kind of foods are good and what kind is not healthy, keep your meals under the scrutiny of your eye so that you know how much calorie is being consumed and remain consistent and motivated to make the seventeen day plan into year long. Many people do make diet plan which has a very good combination of food but they do not know how to carry that practically. That is when the principles come which step by step tell you what should be done and how the plan should be carried.

This would lead to you being healthy. Such people are very active, feel good and enjoy every aspect of life. They are able to take work stress and pressure more easily than the others because their bodies are functioning the way they should. Even doctors encourage the people to maintain the weight according to their height as obese or being fat causes many diseases and problems as you grow old, even bones cannot bear the heavy weight of the body. So living a healthy life and following a good diet plan will lead to immense advantages one can imagine.

# Chapter 4. Benefits of The 17 Day Diet Plan

The main concern these days is of the authentication of the diet plans which are thrown at people haphazardly on the internet. They do not know whom to listen and what not to do. Well, there is good news for them which is that this diet plan is made by the specialist medical doctor who is an expert in weight loss. So there is no doubt in its benefits and authenticity. It basically promotes eating the clean food which means the natural food grown by the farmers. There is nothing artificial involved in it. It is quite realistic as it guides to lose the weight steadily and over a specific period of time. The diet plan is realistic and easy to follow. It does not have any direct health hazards to the people who follow it. The plan is very well organized and it is available to everyone.

The best thing about this plan is that it promotes the exercise which is not done by many other diet plan who only focuses on the consumption of food. It is a known and proven fact that exercise is very important for a healthy body. That is why many people these days are joining gym to stay fit. You can get its book which has a lot of detail in it and it can clear any ambiguities regarding the diet. Even vegetarians can follow it as it is not restricted to non-vegetarians only. Even people suffering from diabetes of type I and type II can easily follow it without upsetting their sugar level. Only one time investment is required if you want to buy the book otherwise information regarding this plan is also available on the internet. The diet plan and type of food included in it is not rigid. It can be made flexible according to the need and taste of various individuals.

# Chapter 5. Food to Eat and Foods to Avoid

**Foods to Eat**

_ Citrus fruit are rich in vitamins which are considered the powerhouse that keeps body healthy and fit.

_ Black, kidney, white and garbanzo beans are source of protein and fiber without any saturated fats. They help in slimming the body.

_ Oats have a lot fiber which makes you full without adding any extra weight to the body.

_ White meat such as fish has many benefits and it has less fats so it is a very good substitute for the red meat which is high in fat as compared to white meat.

_ Blueberries have antiaging effect and it gives full filling feeling containing good amount of fiber.

_ Vegetables are very healthy to eat and they do not add any amount of extra weight to the body so consume vegetables more than the meat.

_ Brown rice have large quantity of fiber which makes it the healthier choice. It helps to increase the metabolism and burn fats.

_ Almonds help to reduce weight as they contain healthy fats which do not increase the weight.

_ Green tea has many benefits. It works like water i.e. keeps you hydrated. It helps to increase the metabolism. It also helps in burning of fat and calorie.

_ Lentils provide the fiber and satiating proteins. This also helps to increase the metabolism and burn fats.

_ Eggs have misconception associated with them that they cause weight gain, the reality is quite contrary to it. It is rich in proteins and its intake in breakfast actually helps to reduce weight according to a study.

_ Pine nuts have fatty acids which play an important role in burning the fat and satisfying the hunger at the same time.

_ Low fat milk contains calcium which is the building block of bones so never skip it. It also has fatty acids.

_ Pearl barley are also known by chickpeas. They are good source of fiber, proteins, starch and healthy fats.

_ Quinoa is good to deal with hunger pangs as it gives you wholesome feeling plus it also helps to avoid eating too much.


**Food to Avoid**

_Do not eat the food with high fats in it such as cheese, smoothies, chocolates etc.

_Avoid eating from the fast food restaurants as they lead to weight gain immensely.

_Do not eat cakes and other food which has butter in large quantity.

_Do not eat food that is fried as it contains oil.

_Processed food is also not recommended for eating.

_Junk food of any sort such as chips, biscuits, candies are to be avoided.

_Cut down the usage of sweets and desserts.

_Any type of food which goes against the diet plan should be avoided.

# Chapter 6. Food Plan

Cycle 1

_In the breakfast eat berries with low-fat yoghurt and drink green tea.

_During lunch eat salad with the fresh vegetables you like such as tomatoes, cucumber etc. along with the green tea.

_In the dinner eat salmon with steamed vegetables of your own choice and green tea.

_If you want to take snacks in between then eat sugar free flavored yoghurt.

Cycle 2

_In the breakfast eat seasonal fruit preferably half grape fruit, scrambled eggs without the yolk and green tea.

_During lunch eat spinach salad including tomatoes, homemade vinaigrette and green tea.

_In the dinner take grilled turkey with salad and green tea.

_For the snacks you can take berries with low fat yoghurt

Cycle 3

_In the breakfast you can take cereals with high fiber content with skimmed milk along with green tea.

_During lunch eat pita consisting of whole wheat with lettuce, vegetables such as tomato, carrots and green tea.

_For snacks you can eat the fruits and ice cream sandwich of Skinny Cow

Cycle 4

In this cycle you can repeat the schedule mentioned above as the purpose of this stage is to maintain the weight.

# Chapter 7. Recipes

## Arugula Salad with Watermelon

Ingredients

_two cups of fresh arugula

_one cup watermelon cut into cubes

_ten mint leaves coarsely cut

_two tablespoon feta cheese

Preparation

Put the arugula leaves in a bowl then add watermelon, mint leaves and feta cheese over it. Eat it with your favorite dressing.

## Apple and Carrot Soup

Ingredients

_one onion

_two table spoon olive oil

_one tablespoon chopped garlic

_two apples peeled and chopped

_four carrots cut into ¼ inch pieces

_four cups of low sodium, non-fat vegetable broth

_one teaspoon of your favorite spice

_pepper and salt according to taste

_for garnish, chopped parsley or chives

Preparation

Put olive oil in a deep pan and heat olive oil in it. Then add chopped onion and garlic till they become soft. After four minutes add the carrots and apple and cook them for two minutes. Put the broth in the pan along with cumin and cook till they start boiling. Then lower the heat till they simmer and keep on cooking till the carrots and apples become soft. It will take from fifteen to twenty minutes. Take it off the heat and serve it with the garnishing of parsley or chives along with the salt and pepper of your own choice.

**Creamy White Bean Veggie Dip**

Ingredients

_fifteen ounce cannellini beans, rinsed and drained

_two cloves of garlic

_three tablespoon non-fat yoghurt

_one tablespoon olive oil

_ ¼ cup fresh dill

_three tablespoon lemon juice

__pepper and according to the taste

_dill sprigs for garnishing


Preparation

Put the beans, oil, yoghurt, garlic, lemon juice and dill in a food processor and keep on blending till you get it smooth. Then garnish it with dill. You can serve it with different kind of vegetables such as carrots, cucumber etc.


**Slimming Soup**


Ingredients

_three cups of chopped cabbage

_two yellow chopped squashes

_one chopped onion

_three chopped, large celery stalk

_fifteen ounce of crushed tomatoes

_fourteen ounce of can of fat free chicken broth

_three teaspoons of salt

_one cup vegetable soup

_ ¼ teaspoon of pepper

Preparation

Take a deep, medium sized pan, put the onions, squashes, celery stalks, crushed tomatoes, fat-free chicken broth, salt, pepper and vegetable soup in it. Mix it properly so that all the ingredients are properly blended. Cook it over the medium heat. It will take thirty to forty minutes to make it. Check if the vegetables have become soft, if not, then keep on cooking. When the broth starts to boil then low the heat further till it starts to simmer. This can be refrigerated for further use in the future. You can do the garnishing of your own choice for the taste.

# Conclusion

It has been seen that many people want to lose their extra fats but they lack the right direction. This can now easily be achieved from the given plan above. This kind of diet is very good for large number of population as it is easy to follow and maintain over a period of time. It precisely describes what should be done. All kinds of details are given so that people do not face any problem while following it. Even the recipes are available which helps a lot as now people can cook the meals that go with their diet plan. The type of food used in cooking is easily available and the best thing about it is that it not expensive to buy those ingredients and they are mostly those that are present in our kitchen.

Previously losing weight was a dream of many but it is becoming a reality now. Many people had to suffer because the dieting plan they followed was not composed or made by any proper dietician or nutritionist. They followed the random plans available on the internet or what some friends and family told them. One thing which they did not realized was that what was good for them might not work them so they had to face problems.

With the introduction of 17 Day diet plan the problem of many people has solved. It has become common and it has been widespread in many areas now. People find it easy and healthy to follow. Many have seen the changes in them as it has proven to help them lose the extra weight and achieve their dream weight. The trust in this plan is increasing and there are many followers of this plan. It will be seen in the upcoming years that it is a very good plan to follow. If you want to reduce weight and live a healthy life then this plan has been made for you.

## Thank You Page

I want to personally thank you for reading my book. I hope you found information in this book useful and I would be very grateful if you could leave your honest review about this book. I certainly want to thank you in advance for doing this.

If you have the time, you can check my other books too.

CPSIA information can be obtained at www.ICGtesting.com
Printed in the USA
BVOW01s0331220916

462824BV00008B/183/P

9 781682 120491